AF772414

Neck Care

Second Edition

How to Relieve and Prevent Pain from Neck Problems

Editor:
Andrew Cole, MD
Clinical Assistant Professor, Department of Physical Medicine and Rehabilitation, University of Washington School of Medicine. Medical Director, The Spine Center, Overlake Hospital Medical Center, Bellevue, Washington. Practicing at Northwest Spine and Sports Physicians, PC, Bellevue, Washington.

Consultant:
Cary C. Bucko, PT
Director, The Spine Center, Overlake Hospital Medical Center, Bellevue, Washington.

Additional Participants:
Jeffrey K. Pearson, DO, Consultant
Martin Bilger, PhD, Research Editor
Murray A. Swanson, BS, Publisher's General Editor

First Edition Author:
Kenneth B. Washburn, MD

Copyright © 1999
Medic Publishing Co.
P.O. Box 943, Issaquah, WA 98027-0035
Voice 425-222-0844 Fax 425-222-0845
All Rights Reserved

Contents

Introduction 3

Part I—Measures Physicians May Prescribe

- Cold 4
- Heat 4
- Massage 5
- Immobilization 5
- Rest 5
- Neck Exercises
  - Isometric Exercises 6
  - Mobilizing Exercises 8
  - Base-of-neck Exercises 9
- Relaxing the Upper Neck 10
- Traction 11
- Other Treatments 12

Part II—Protection and Prevention

- Spinal Posture 13
- Head Posture 14
- Posture Illustrations 14
- Relaxation 21
- Fitness 23

Caution

This booklet is intended to supplement your physician's care. If there is a conflict between what your physician says and what you read in this booklet, follow your physician's advice. Only a physician is qualified to fully evaluate your neck pain.

Once under a doctor's care, it is important to continue under that care. Contact your physician promptly if improvement does not occur as anticipated or if new symptoms appear.

Introduction

The neck (cervical spine) is amazing. It bends and rotates, carries a heavy weight (your head may weigh 10 pounds or more), and protects vital nerves and blood vessels. The neck is supported and moved by a complex system of ligaments and muscles, and, like the lower back, it may cause pain. Most problems fall into three categories:

- **Age-related degeneration.** Changes in neck **joints** can be seen in X-rays of almost everyone over 40 years of age. **Discs**, the cushions between vertebrae, dry out and shrink. Bony projections, called **spurs** or osteophytes, may form. The openings in vertebrae where nerves pass through become narrowed—**foraminal stenosis**. Narrowing may also occur in the central canal that surrounds the spinal cord—**central stenosis.** These changes sometimes cause symptoms.

- **Sudden injury (trauma)**. A typical neck injury may be caused by sudden and forceful bending. In auto accidents, this bending first in one direction and then in the other at high velocity is called **whiplash.** Similar bending beyond normal range also occurs in sports and falls. The actual injury is usually an overstretching or slight tearing of soft tissues (muscles, ligaments, tendons), which is called a **strain** or **sprain**. Most injuries like these are mild and heal quickly, often in two weeks or so. If the tearing is more severe or if other structures are injured, healing will take longer, but *about two-thirds of all trauma patients recover in two months or less*. The rest, with few exceptions, also become pain free eventually, although some people will have occasional neck pain throughout their lives.

- **Postural neck syndrome.** This is mostly a problem of position that causes the neck to be stiff and painful. It is common among people who work at a desk or bench. It also happens in activities or jobs that require awkward positions—plumbing and painting, for example. Ordinary **stress** may also lead to this kind of neck problem.

Whatever the cause, there are a number of things you can do to relieve or eliminate your pain. Be aware, however, that some of the instructions in this booklet may not be right for you. Follow your doctor's orders and heed the "caution" on the previous page.

Part I—Measures Physicians May Prescribe

COLD

Ice packs are usually recommended for the first 48 to 72 hours (two to three days) after a soft tissue injury. Ice decreases inflammation, swelling, and pain. Ice also helps relieve muscle spasm during this early period and at any time thereafter. You can purchase a cervical ice pack or make your own. Gel-filled packs that will still conform to your neck when frozen are probably the easiest to use, but you can make your own pack from crushed ice in a plastic bag wrapped with a towel. *Apply up to 20 minutes, only to back or sides of neck.* Do this every hour if your schedule permits, but even three or four times a day should help.

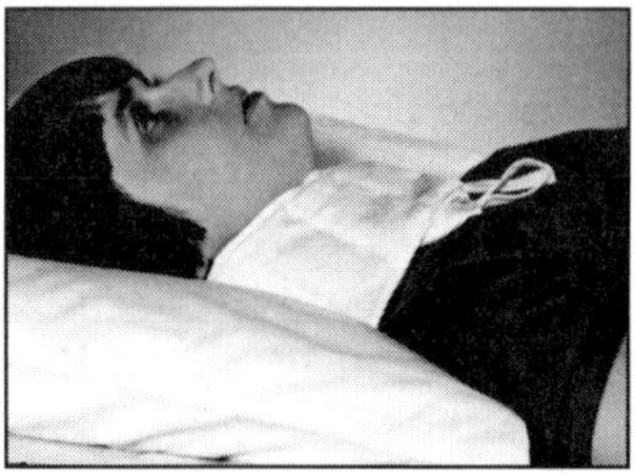

A cervical pack from a hospital supply firm applies moist heat or cold.

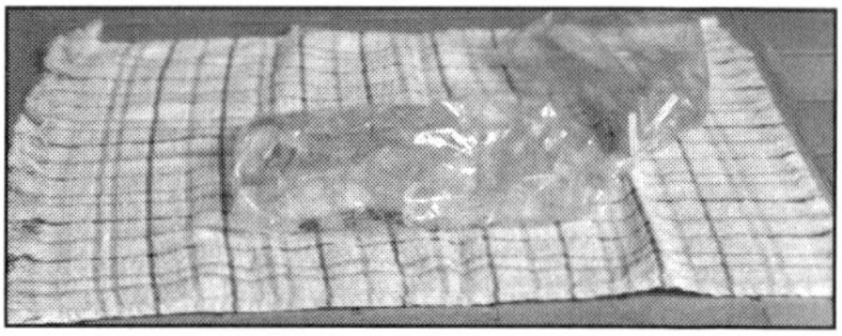

Use a towel for frostbite protection.

Caution: Be careful to avoid freezing your skin. Also, some people are very sensitive to cold objects on their skin. Check with your doctor.

HEAT

Heat is often useful for pain *after* cold treatment, that is, after about three days. It relieves pain and muscle spasm. Be careful to use it only for brief periods—not more than 15 to 20 minutes at a time. Wait at least 1 hour between applications. Heat treatment works by improving the blood supply, but *don't overdo it.* Prolonged heat treatment might make the symptoms worse.

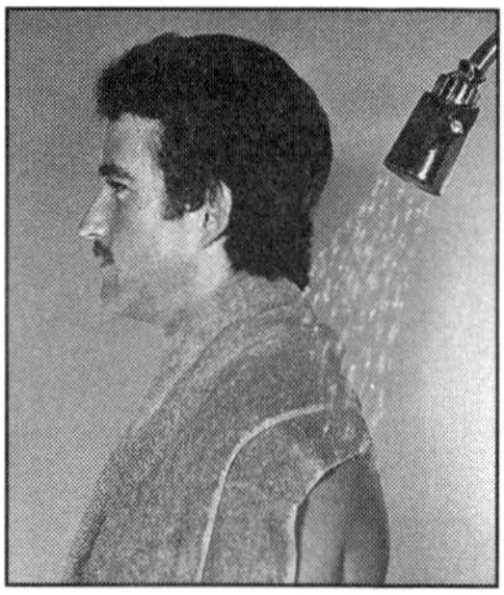

Try up to 10 minutes in a hot shower with a towel.

Heat is helpful before exercises or traction. A hot shower, hot pad, or whirlpool helps to relax muscles and make the exercises or traction more effective. (See page 11 for one type of traction.)

Electric heating pads should never be used while you are asleep. Even low heat for prolonged periods can cause serious burns.

MASSAGE

Although it doesn't treat the underlying problem, gentle massage, up to 15 minutes, may give temporary relief. Rub and squeeze your neck in ways that feel comfortable. For lubrication, use a lotion or oil. Avoid pushing or pulling—leave this to a trained professional.

IMMOBILIZATION

Sometimes following a neck sprain and for other specific problems, your doctor may prescribe a cervical collar. In some cases, when the doctor wants no movement at all, a rigid collar is used. Usually, however, a soft collar is ordered. This allows limited movement while providing some support, relaxation, and warmth. If you wear a collar, follow your doctor's instruction and these rules:

1. **Get a good fit.** Be sure your *chin is not raised and your head not pushed forward.* To get a better fit, your physician might ask you to try the collar with the closure in the front.
2. **Limit use.** Discontinue as soon as directed. Prolonged use leads to stiff joints and muscle wasting. Remove for short periods at first and then for longer periods.
3. **Possibly use in bed.** A soft collar might be helpful while you sleep.
4. **Watch for problems.** If discomfort from the collar develops, call your doctor or physical therapist.

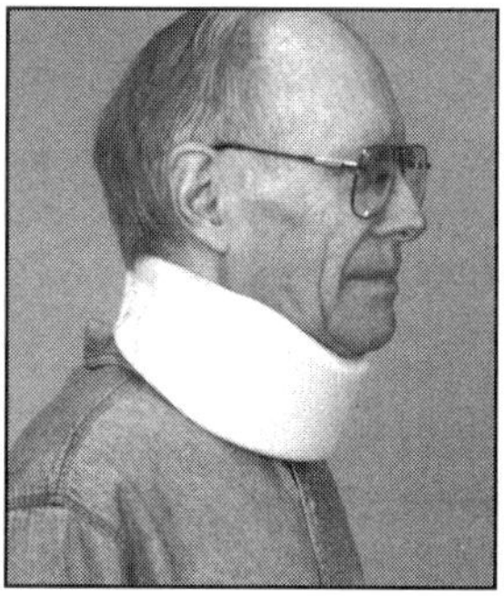

Collar courtesy Allcare Medical

A soft collar should fit comfortably with your head level.

REST

If strain is causing a lot of pain, you might have to quit most activities for a few days. Doctors sometimes order bed rest because walking, standing, and even sitting require strained muscles to continue to work. They must support and control the head. A proper reclining position (see page 19) gives muscles a better opportunity to recover, but don't overdo it. *Rest only as long as necessary—prolonged rest delays recovery; gradual use speeds recovery.*

While in bed, gentle neck motion might help. Support your neck and head with a soft pillow and roll your head from side to side within your pain tolerance. Do this no more than 1 to 2 minutes at a time.

ISOMETRIC NECK EXERCISES

> **Caution:** If you have high blood pressure (hypertension), check with your doctor before doing isometric exercises.

Isometric exercises strengthen muscles *without movement.* They also tend to relax tense muscles. There is less risk of strain or injury than with other kinds of exercise.

Follow these guidelines:

1. **Begin only with your physician's approval.** Do not begin while you still have severe pain.
2. **Start slowly and work up.** Begin by doing 3 repetitions of each exercise 3 times a day. Every day or so add a repetition until you are doing 8 to 10 repetitions each time.
3. **Push moderately.** Push as hard as you can *without causing pain.*
4. **Breathe out as you push.** Holding your breath during these exercises tends to raise blood pressure. Exhale *slowly* while you are pushing.
5. **Relax between contractions.** Concentrate on relaxing. This is necessary to get the full benefit from these exercises.
6. **Stop if pain increases.**

Isometric Exercise 1
Resisted Extension

Clasp your hands behind your head (not your neck). Tuck in your chin. Push your head firmly into your hands while using your hands to prevent movement. Hold for a slow count of 5 while exhaling slowly. Then concentrate on relaxing a few moments before repeating.

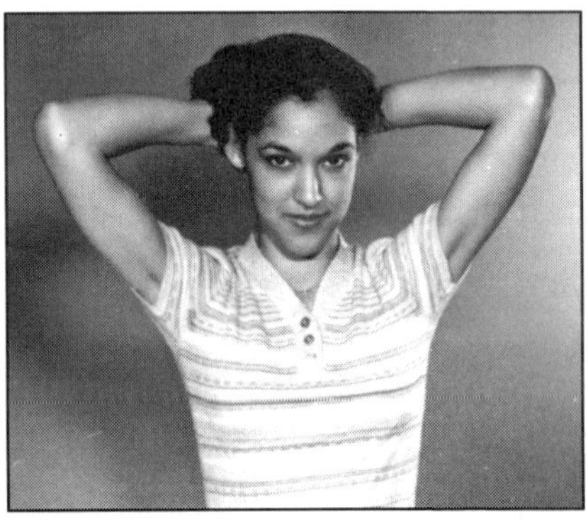

Isometric Exercise 2
Resisted Flexion

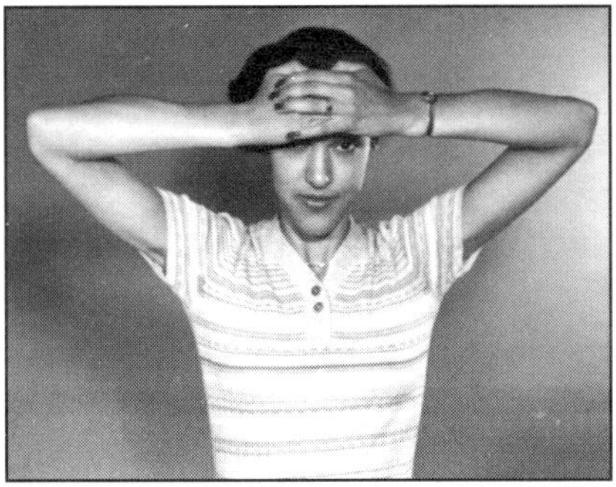

Place your hands on your forehead (one hand on top of the other). Tuck in your chin. Push your head into your hands, using your hands to prevent movement. Hold for a slow count of 5 while exhaling slowly. Concentrate on relaxing, and then repeat.

Isometric Exercise 3
Resisted Side-bend

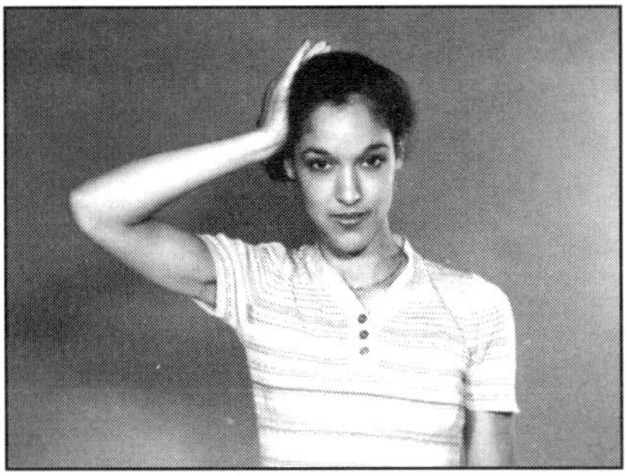

Place your right hand above your right ear. Push and hold for a slow count of 5 while exhaling slowly. Relax and then repeat. Keep your head straight and level.

Repeat with your left hand above your left ear.

Isometric Exercise 4
Resisted Rotation

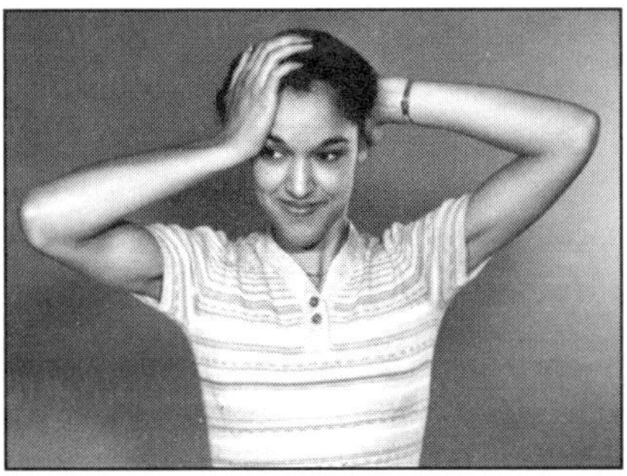

Place your right hand on your right temple and your left hand at the left-rear of your head. Your hands will be diagonally opposite. Look to your right and push into your hands as if to turn your head. Keep your head straight and level. Hold for a slow count of 5 while exhaling slowly. Relax, and then repeat.

Repeat with your hands reversed, looking left.

MOBILIZATION EXERCISES

Caution: If you have rheumatoid arthritis or have had a neck fracture in the last year, do not do mobilization exercises.

When your doctor permits more-or-less normal movement, do the following 3 times a day. If they cause pain, stop and do only isometric exercises (pages 6 and 7). Snaps and pops are common and are no reason to stop unless they are associated with pain.

These exercises, using gradually increasing distance as tolerated, will, in most people, speed the recovery time after an injury.

Mobilization 1: Rotation

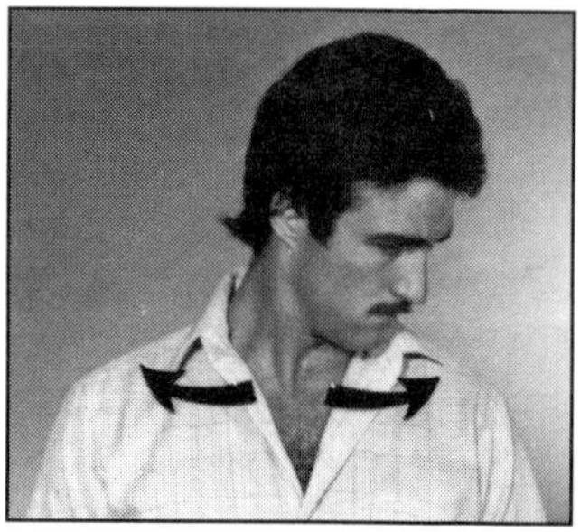

Nod your head slightly downward, your chin toward your chest. Slowly move your chin toward one shoulder *as far as is comfortable,* and then toward the other shoulder. Keep your chin tucked and do not try for extra distance by stretching or forcing your neck. *Additional distance will come gradually.* Do 5 to 10 times.

Mobilization 2: Side Bend

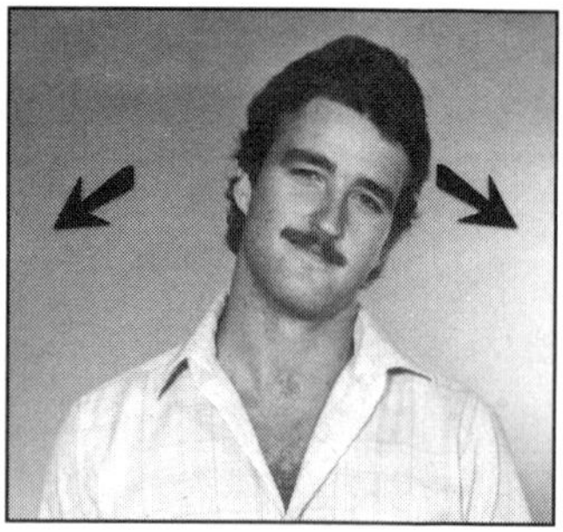

Tilt your head slowly first to one side and then toward the other *as far as is comfortable.* Do not allow your head to tilt backward and do not stretch or force your neck for extra distance. Do 5 to 10 times.

Mobilization 3: Flexion

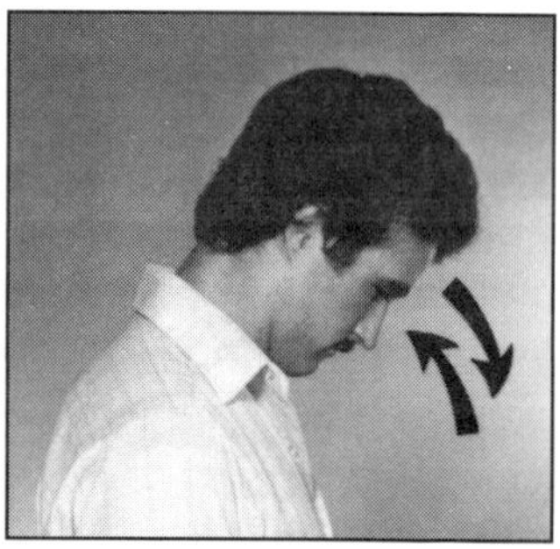

Slowly lower your head, your chin toward your chest. Return to your beginning position. Do not tilt your head backward and do not stretch or force your neck. Do 5 to 10 times.

EXERCISES FOR THE BASE OF THE NECK

Tension in the muscles around the base of the neck often causes pain and discomfort. The tension may be due to other neck problems or simply to neck posture or holding one position too long. These two exercises usually give relief. They may be done 2 or 3 times a day or more often if needed.

Shoulder Circles

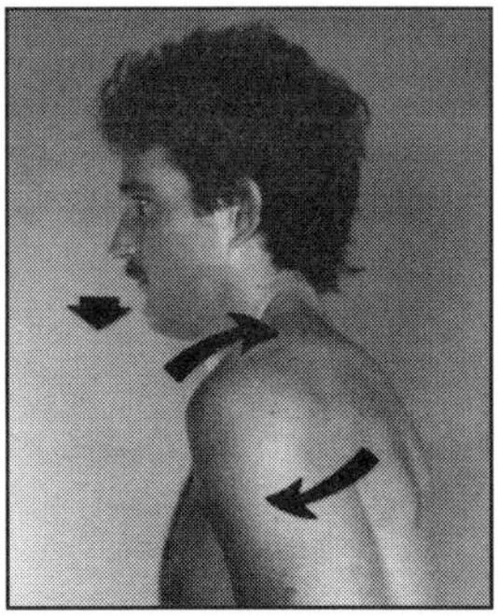

Stand straight and tall, your chin tucked in, your arms relaxed. Move both of your shoulders in small circles by first raising them slightly and then moving them backward, down, forward, and around. Do not attempt to make as large a circle as possible—stay within your comfort range. Begin with 5 to 10 repetitions, gradually adding repetitions until you are doing 20 circles.

Shoulder-Blade Squeeze

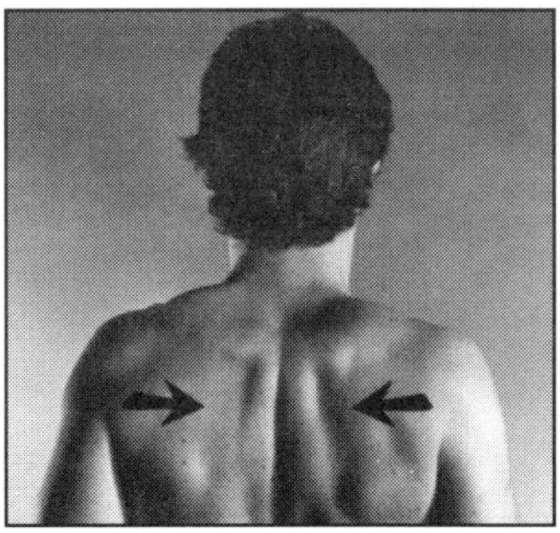

Stand straight and tall *in front of a mirror,* your chin tucked in, your arms relaxed. Push your shoulder blades back as close together as you can while keeping your shoulders from rising (check in mirror). Return to your starting position. Concentrate on relaxing a few moments before repeating the exercise. Repeat 5 times in the beginning. Gradually add repetitions until you are doing 15 squeezes.

RELAXING THE UPPER NECK

Tension at the top of the neck, like tension elsewhere in the neck, may come from holding a bent position too long. This can happen with desk work or occupations that require an awkward head position. It also happens from watching television while lying down with the head propped up.

Sometimes the uppermost joints lock. This is where the base of the skull connects to the first neck vertebra (atlas). Motion is then restricted. Tenderness, inflammation, and pain follow; headache is common. This condition is called *occipital* (back of head) *cephalgia* (headache).

Physical therapists and other practitioners may be able to mobilize the locked joints by gentle stretching and other movement. You can also do the following at home.

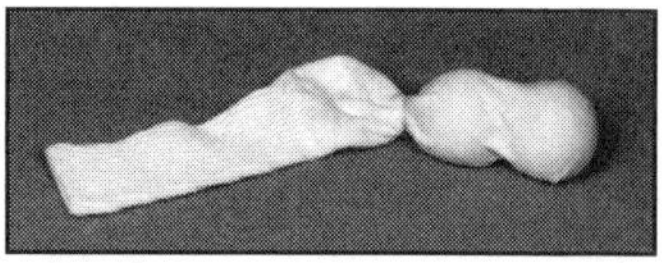

Place 2 tennis balls in a sock. Use a twist tie or rubber band to hold the balls in the toe.

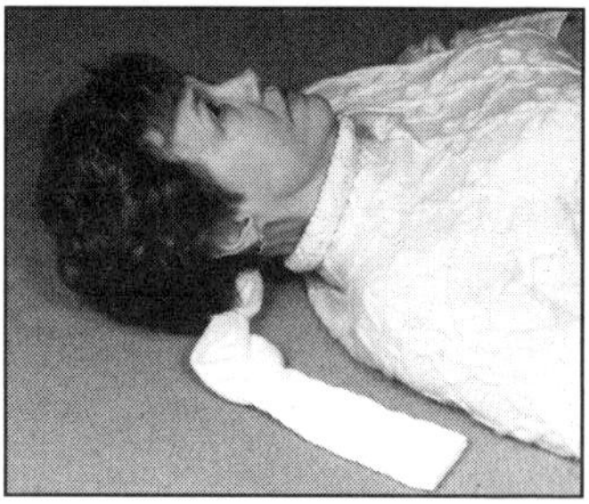

Lie on a carpeted floor. Run your fingers behind your ears, over the bony ridges and into the depressions beyond the ridges. Place the tennis balls into these depressions (occipital condyles) and lie this way until the surrounding muscles relax. *Take care that the balls do not slip down under your neck. Keeping your chin down should prevent this.* If it doesn't, place a small towel at the lower edge of the balls. Expect relaxation to begin within 10 minutes or so, but there is no time limit as long as you are comfortable.

Important

Although neck exercises can be very helpful for tension and other problems, long-term relief requires attention to posture and other habits. Part II, which begins on page 13, covers these areas.

TRACTION

> *Caution:* Traction helps in many cases but is not for everyone. Exceptions include those with rheumatoid neck disease or with muscle weakness in trunk and arms. Referral to a physical therapist for instruction will help to avoid injury. Horizontal (recumbant) traction might also be considered.

If your doctor orders home traction, buy only the kit that the doctor or staff specifies. It will have a head harness that pulls almost entirely on the base of the skull, with little pull on the chin. The front piece will fit over the point of the chin, not under the chin.

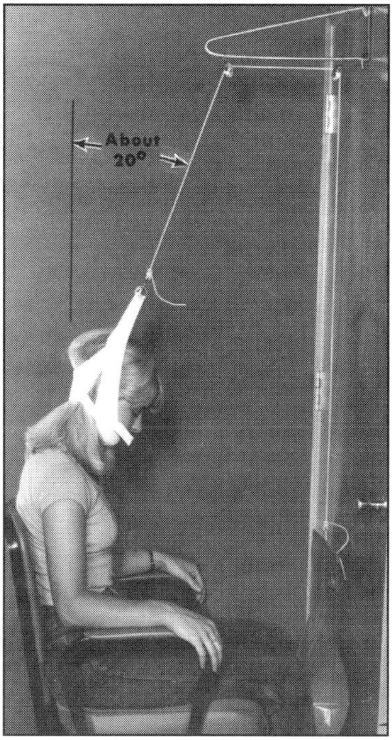

1. **Choose a door in a quiet place.** Have a helper nearby.
2. **Fill weight bag according to doctor's order.** The plastic type is marked for water. Five to 10 pounds is common, but more may be ordered.
3. **Select a chair with firm support** for your lower back. Place it *facing* the door. Sit with your back against the chair. Support your arms on armrests or a pillow.
4. **Make sure the head harness fits properly**—over the point of your chin with *almost all pull on the base of your skull.* Straps between front and rear should not press on neck.
5. **Check the forward angle of your head**—about 20 degrees. This angle usually occurs when your knees almost touch the door.
6. **Start with the weight bag on your lap** and the rope slightly slack. Gradually ease the bag off of your lap. *You must control the bag so that it does not drop suddenly.*
7. **Continue as long as directed,** perhaps up to 20 minutes. For intermittent traction, rest occasionally with the bag in your lap.

Typically the order is for 2 sessions a day, but if pain is severe, more may be suggested. If you get no relief in 1 or 2 weeks or if traction increases your pain, consult your doctor.

OTHER TREATMENTS

Physical Therapy. Physical therapists treat injury or disease by non-drug measures such as exercise, mobilization of joints and soft tissues, light, electrotherapy, hydrotherapy, heat and cold. Their objectives are to reduce pain and speed your return to normal function and strength. They will apply the best methods for your situation. *Physical therapists are also excellent teachers, able to instruct you in exercises and in ways to avoid injury on your job and in daily activities.* Treatments by a physical therapist might include:

> **Deep heat.** Ultrasound treatments have deep heating effects which decrease pain, increase muscle flexibility, and remove the byproducts of inflammation.
>
> **TENS.** Transcutaneous electrical stimulation (TENS) may relieve chronic pain. TENS units can also be rented for home use.

Manipulation or mobilization. This approach is intended to improve range of motion and to decrease pain. It is performed by osteopaths (DO), chiropractors (DC), physical therapists (PT), and sometimes by MDs. Various techniques are used.

Medication. NSAIDs—nonsteroidal antiinflammatory drugs—either in over-the-counter or prescription strength, are most commonly used for strains and sprains. Other pain relievers (analgesics), such as acetaminophen, may be used. Muscle relaxants and antidepressants are sometimes given. For extreme pain, a short period of narcotic analgesic may be used. Your doctor and/or pharmacist should inform you about possible side effects of any prescribed medication. Medications should be taken exactly as prescribed, and suspicion of a problem with them reported promptly.

Trigger point injections. Sometimes a patient has very painful muscle spasms, which may be helped by an injection into the muscle. The injection may relax the muscle.

Acupuncture. This ancient treatment, in which needles are inserted into exact locations, is sometimes helpful.

Part II—Protection and Prevention

SPINAL POSTURE
Developing the Tall Position

Drooping shoulders lead to neck strain because the head must be tilted back to compensate. To correct the tendency toward drooping shoulders, learn to *stand tall, sit tall,* and *walk tall.*

Imagine making your body as long as possible. Consider yourself a *marionette on a string* pulling your head up with your knees slightly bent. Keep your head high, your chin slightly tucked in, and your abdominal muscles pulled in.

> **Caution:** Avoid the military posture of "chin up and chest out." Keep chin down. Do not arch your lower back.

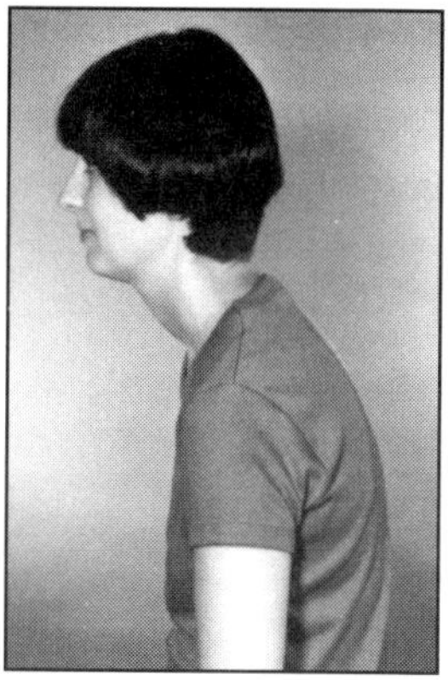
When shoulders droop, the backward curve in the neck increases, causing strain.

Take time out to be tall. If your work requires you to lean forward for periods of time, pause frequently, relax, breathe deeply and stretch your body into the tall position. Use the stretching exercises on pages 8 and 9.

Check the curve in your lower back. Your lumbar curve may contribute to neck strain. The curves in your lower and upper back work together to keep your body balanced. If your lower back curves inward more than slightly, your upper back will tend to curve outward more than slightly. To develop a tall posture, you may have to work on reducing the curve in your lower back.

Back exercises help. You can correct an excessive lower back curve by regularly doing some simple and easy exercises that strengthen and stretch muscles attached to the pelvis. Such exercises are described in ***Back Care,*** a companion booklet dealing with the lower back.

Large-breasted women take note: The weight of your breasts tends to pull your shoulders down and forward. If you make tall posture a habit, you may avoid neck strain. Extremely large-breasted women might consider reduction mammaplasty (surgery). A study showed it relieved neck strain in a majority of cases.

HEAD POSTURE

The position of your head and neck in your daily activities may cause strain. As much as is practical, *aim to keep your head in a neutral position, balanced over your shoulders.*

Most importantly:

- **Avoid tilting your head backward.** Avoid tilting it back *slightly* for a *long period.* Avoid tilting it *far back* even for a *short period.*
- **Avoid holding your head forward** against gravity for a long period, such as when reading or writing. Take frequent breaks.

In general, avoid *extreme positions.* Don't look over your shoulder. Turn your body instead. Avoid tilting your head far to one side.

Avoid holding *any one position for a long time,* usually no more than about 15 minutes.

The illustrations which follow show examples of both correct and incorrect positions.

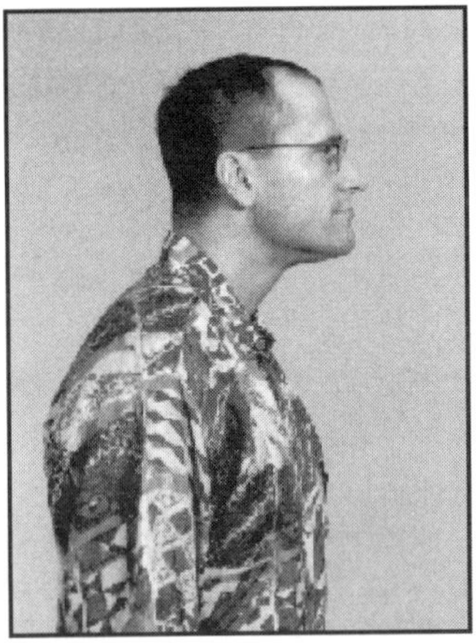

Incorrect. Don't take the "spectator" position—chin up and head forward. This is also known as the "attack" position.

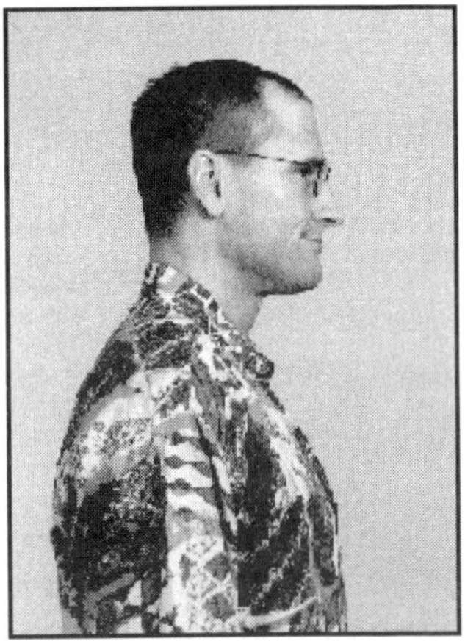

Correct. Keep your chin down. Sit *toward the rear* in theaters and in auditoriums with raised platforms.

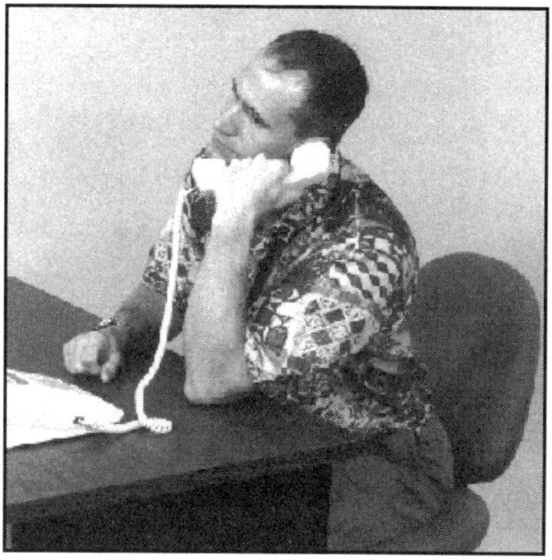

Incorrect. Don't lean over a desk. Don't cradle phone on shoulder or lean into phone.

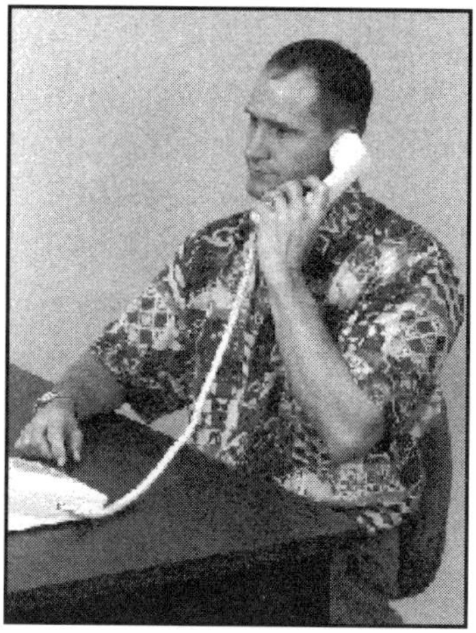

Correct. When seated at a desk, use an upright posture with lower back supported. *If on the phone for long periods, be sure to use a headset.*

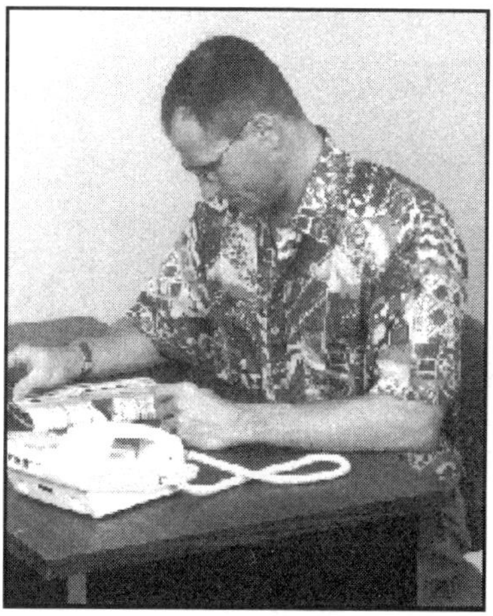

Incorrect. Avoid reading with your head down for a prolonged period.

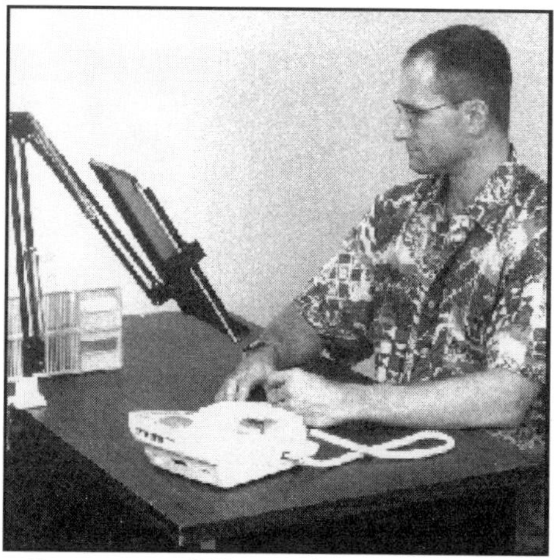

Correct. When doing a lot of reading or other desk work, use a copy holder or study stand to permit an erect head position at least part of the time.

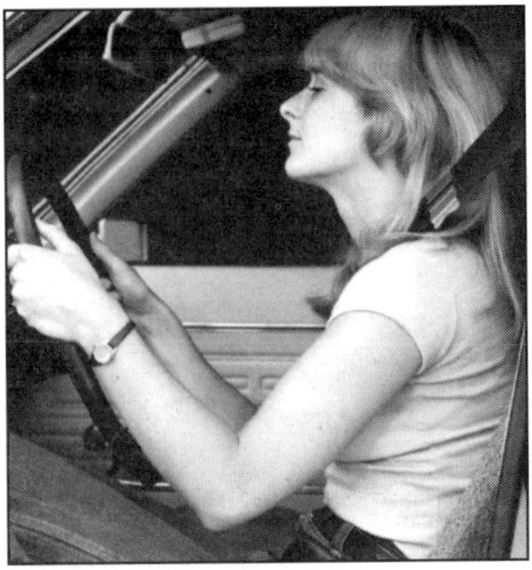

Incorrect. Avoid driving with your chin up, even slightly.

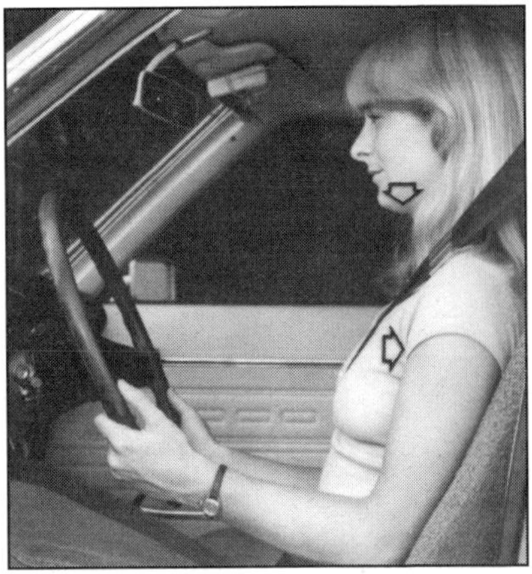

Correct. Adjust seat forward so you can reach the pedals easily. Sit back and keep chin down. Add back support if necessary. When safe to do so, keep hands *low* on steering wheel.

On long trips, stop every hour or so and do exercises such as those on pages 9 and 13.

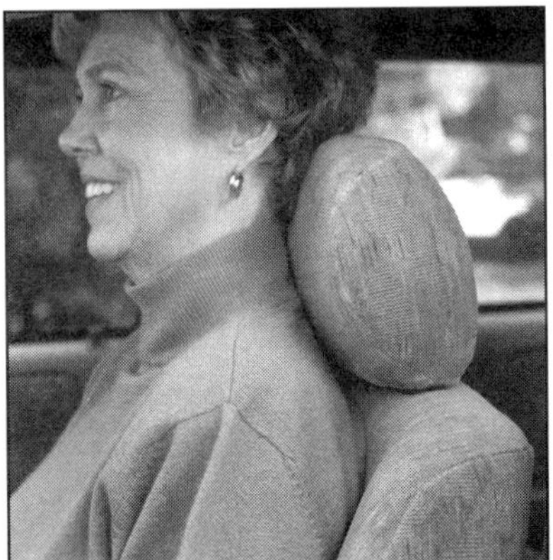

Incorrect. Avoid riding in a vehicle with the head support behind your neck. In this position, the support may worsen injury in an accident.

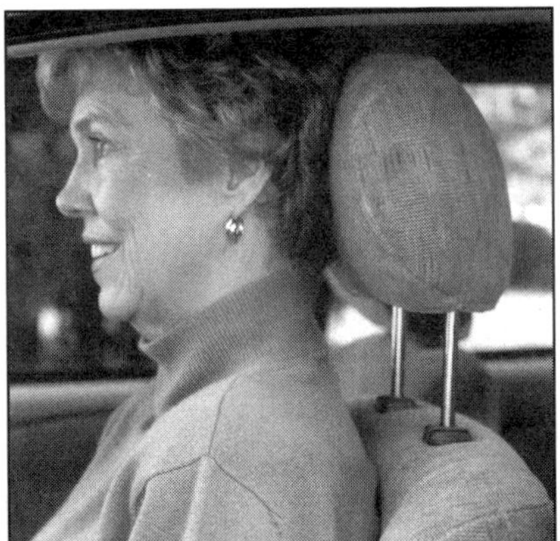

Correct. Raise the support so it is opposite the back of your head.

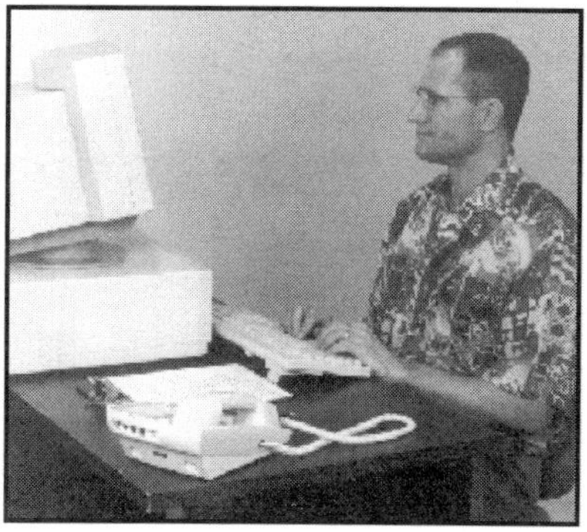

Incorrect. Computer monitor is too high if your chin must be raised, even slightly. Avoid bifocal eyeglasses (see page 20). Avoid continuous keyboard work.

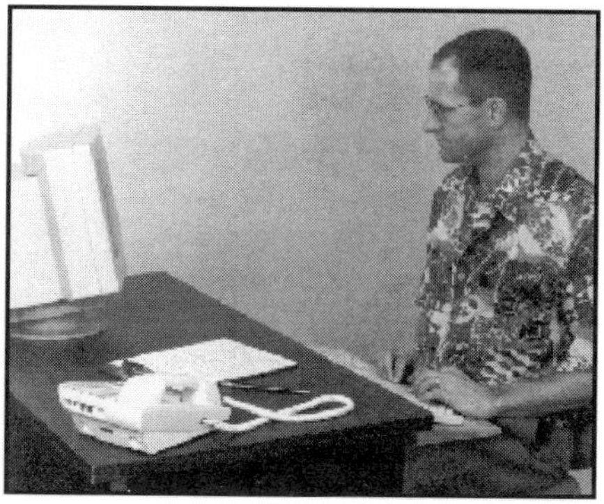

Correct. Monitor directly on desk top usually allows proper viewing—*top of monitor screen slightly below eye level.* Keyboard is best on a tray at lap level. Get up every 20 to 30 minutes and do stretching exercises.

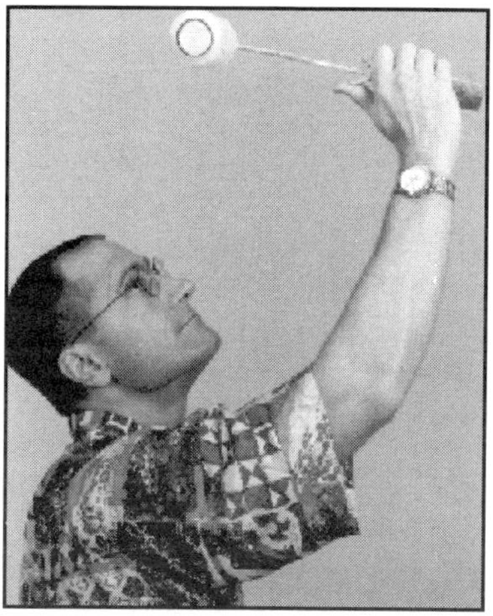

Incorrect. Avoid working over your head such as painting a ceiling while standing on the floor.

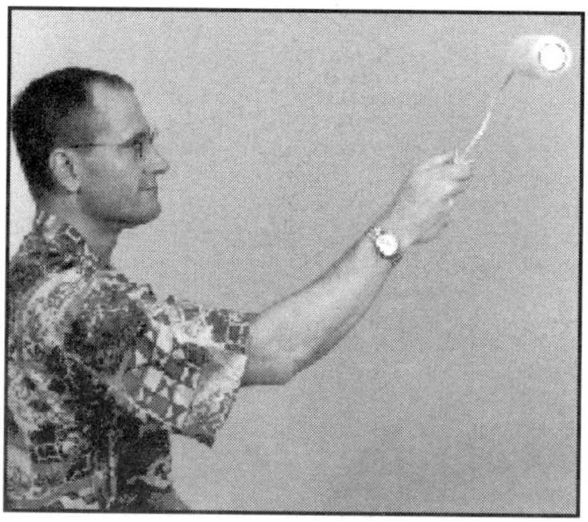

Correct. Use stilts, ladder, or scaffolding when doing any work that would otherwise be above your head.

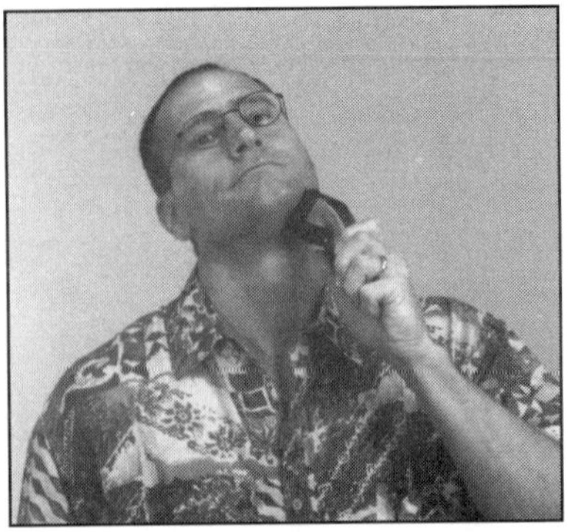

Incorrect. Avoid tilting your head backward while shaving.

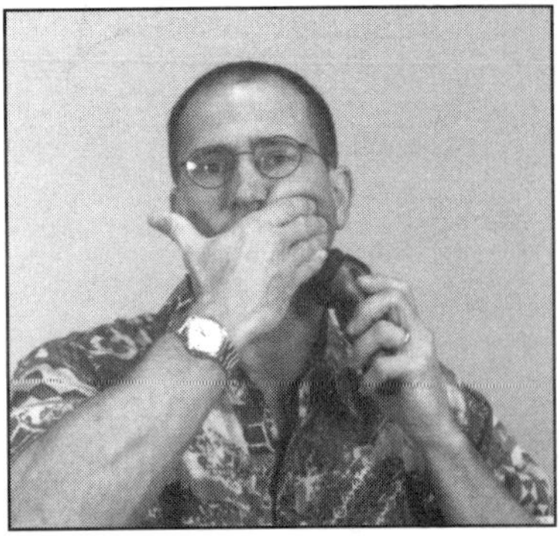

Correct. Stretch skin with hand and keep head close to level.

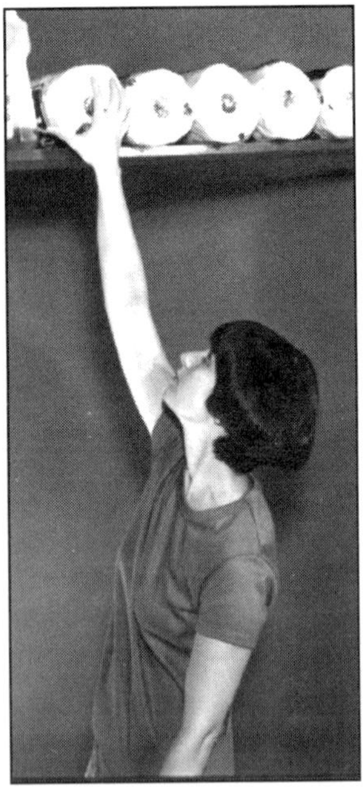

Incorrect. Avoid reaching to high shelves, especially with your head bent to one side or backward.

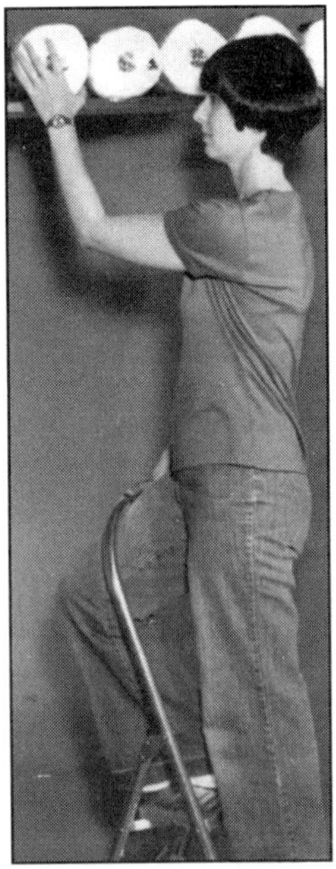

Correct. Keep a folding ladder or step stool in the kitchen or work place and use it for access to high shelves. Store often used items at convenient levels.

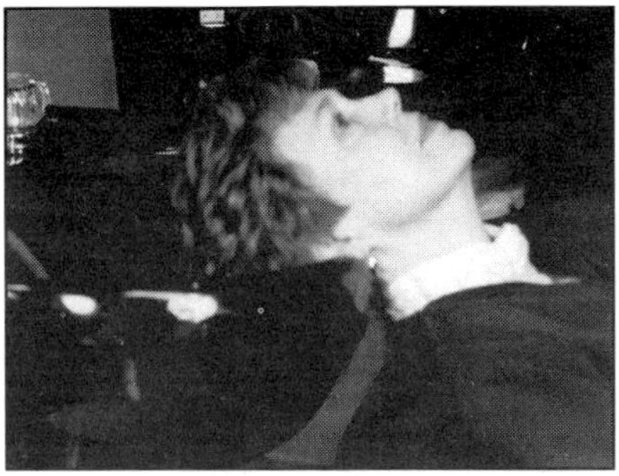

Incorrect. Do not rest your neck on edge of shampoo basin. Apart from the hazard to the neck, the vertebral artery can be pinched, affecting circulation.

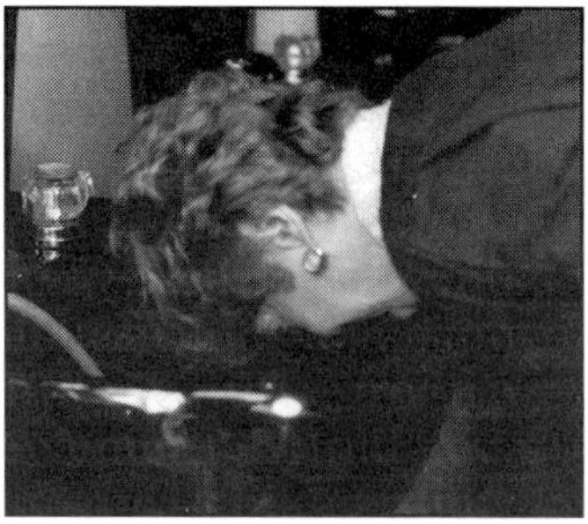

Correct. Wash your hair face down in the basin or use a shower.

Incorrect. When sleeping on your back, your head should not be raised. Do not watch television or read with your head propped up.

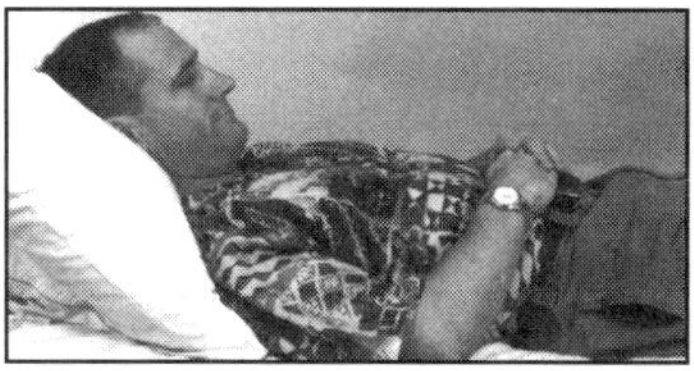

Correct. When sleeping on your back, use a moldable pillow (see next page) that supports your head and neck in a level position. Use large pillows or a roll under your knees.

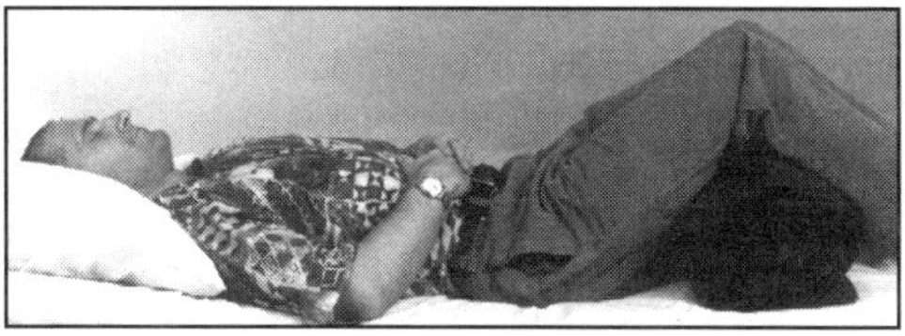

Incorrect. When sleeping on your side, do not allow your head to tilt up or down. Avoid a large or buoyant pillow that raises your head.

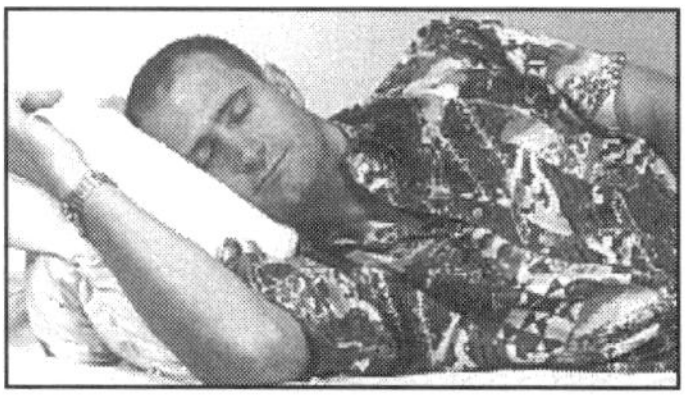

Correct. A pillow should support both head and neck, keeping your head level. Arms should be below neck. See pillow discussion, next page.

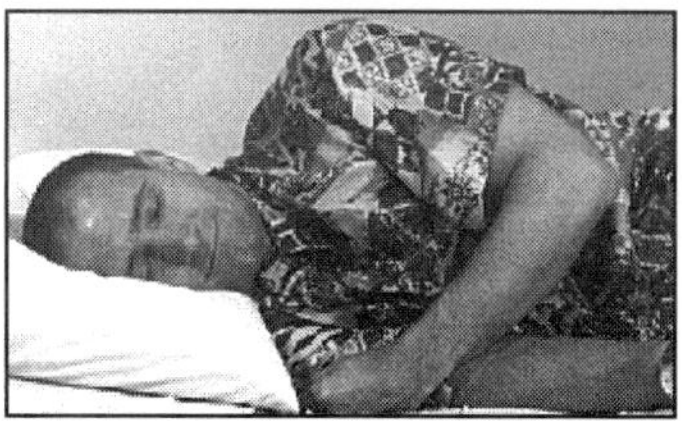

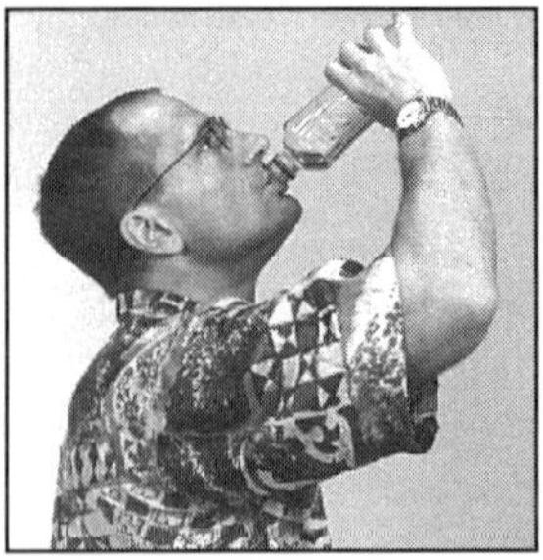

Incorrect. Do not drink directly from a bottle or can.

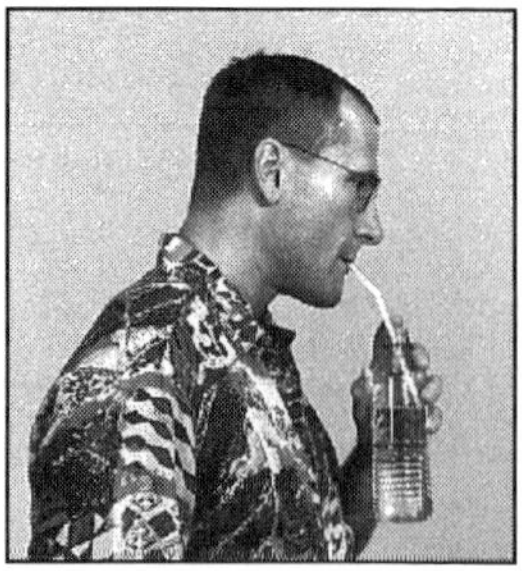

Correct. Use straws or cups.

The pillow problem. You need a comfortable pillow that supports both the head and neck in a level position, but no one type suits everyone. Down fill is often preferred but, like feathers, may be allergenic (special covers are available). Foam may be too buoyant. Polyester pillows vary in design and may or may not be too buoyant. In a Swedish study of special cervical pillows, two out of three people preferred a design of soft polyurethane with raised upper and lower sections, each supported by a firmer core.

The bifocal problem. When looking at objects close-up near eye level, bifocal eyeglasses force you to tilt your head backward. If you are in this situation often, use reading glasses. If your job requires close work above eye level, order bifocals with the reading part at the top of the lens. These are called "meter reader's glasses."

Toting a load. Carrying briefcases, laptop computers, and shoulder bags can cause neck and shoulder pain. A weight on one shoulder puts stress on the other one and on the spine. Repetition makes it worse.

- **Lighten the load.** Find ways to carry less weight.
- **Split the load.** Use two small loads rather than one large one.
- **Switch the load.** Change sides often.
- **Use a day pack.** Adjust the pack so that it does not bounce. Adjust a *heavy* pack so as to put most weight on hips and lower torso.

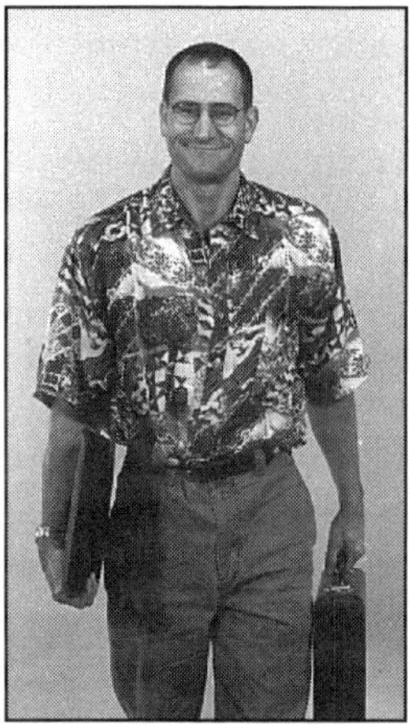

Splitting the load

RELAXATION

Mental stress can have a physical effect. Quite often the neck suffers. Reducing frustration, anger, and anxiety is therefore one of the most important and effective paths to overall health, and, in many cases, to relieving neck strain.

Relaxing, however, is easier said than done. Circumstances may seem impossible—the boss is too demanding, income is too low, expenses are too high, and your spouse doesn't understand. Sometimes circumstances can and should be changed, but even if they stay the same, there are fruitful things you can do. You can (1) work on your mind-set, that is, the way you approach circumstances, and (2) adopt relaxation techniques.

Favorable mind-sets. You can adopt these mind-sets by saying the statements to yourself. You can learn to fulfill the images. As you do so, tension will drop.

1. I am in charge of my responses.
2. I do my best now and do not worry about what might happen later.
3. I do one thing at a time.
4. I say honestly, although graciously, what I feel.
5. I treat everyone, including children, with respect.
6. If I have a sexual problem, I express my feelings to my partner, and I work on the problem.
7. I am not a slave to competition. I do what is right.
8. I realize I am not perfect, and I do not berate myself for my mistakes. I am learning and growing.
9. I take care of my body. I choose to be healthy.

Don't give up because you can't seem to adopt all of these ideas at once. Progress is what counts.

But if you think this mind-set approach is too difficult, take heart—the next instruction, about a relaxation technique, is easy. Follow a few simple steps, and your body will respond by relaxing. It works.

RELAXATION, continued

Meditation is a reliable and effective relaxation technique. It lowers brain wave activity (to alpha) and, when practiced daily, often reduces a host of nervous symptoms. The word *meditation* may or may not have a religious meaning. Its use here means simply an exercise that can help you relax.

There are various ways to meditate. The following way is simple and effective.

1. Sit comfortably, hands in lap, thumb tips touching, eyes closed or focused on some point straight ahead. In the beginning, you may find it easier to lie down.
2. Take a slow, deep breath. Count "1" to yourself while you inhale.
3. Slowly exhale completely, while counting "2" silently.
4. Repeat, counting "3" while inhaling and "4" while exhaling. Continue until you reach the count of "10." Start again at "1."
5. If thoughts come, pay no attention. Let them drift through. Do the same with sounds and other distractions. Your attention should be on breathing, counting, and relaxing your body.

Try this for 5 to 10 minutes in the beginning. 30 minutes a day is ideal, but do what you can. Even 10 minutes is helpful.

Other relaxation techniques include biofeedback and hypnosis. Biofeedback requires training and equipment. Hypnosis can be done by oneself—it works by way of suggestion.

> **What** you do about stress is not as important as doing **something.** Get help. Attend a seminar. Read a book on the subject and follow its recommendations.

FITNESS

Overall fitness requires exercise, proper weight, good diet, control of stress, and other healthy habits. Fitness has many rewards, including a neck less likely to cause pain.

Smoking, for example, can affect the neck by reducing circulation in the small blood vessels that supply the area around the spinal discs. Exercise, on the other hand, increases circulation.

Eat right. Most people need to eat less fat and sugar and more vegetables, fruits, and whole grains. Extra calcium helps reduce age-related osteoporosis (bone softening). Some authorities recommend extra vitamin C to help build the collagen needed by spinal discs. Others believe that 8 glasses of water a day will slow the disc-drying process that comes to everyone with aging.

Control your weight. Extra pounds can contribute to neck problems by causing your spine to sag. Research suggests that weight control may be easier than you think. Talk to your doctor.

Exercise your whole body. Aerobic exercise is rhythmic motion done long enough and hard enough to keep your heart rate in a "target range" for at least 15 minutes. Longer periods, along with a warm-up, are usually recommended. Exercising 5 or 6 days a week is best, but 3 days a week will probably maintain whatever level of fitness you achieve.

Be careful! Heavy exercise can be dangerous. An exercise program requires your doctor's approval and should always be increased gradually in stages. Furthermore, it is not necessary to do any exercise at a strenuous level. Some people should not try for the aerobic target but should just move at a comfortable pace.

The following activities are generally good, but heed the warnings that will be given.

- **Walking**
- **Motorized Treadmill**
- **Bicycling**
- **Jogging**
- **Swimming**

Walking is an excellent, low-risk exercise. It can be done indoors, such as in a shopping mall or on a motorized treadmill at home or in a gym. Work up to at least a half hour per session. Keep your posture tall—no forward slumping. Let your hips swing freely. Use well-cushioned shoes or special shock-absorbing insoles. At least in the beginning, choose only level areas.

A motorized treadmill is the equipment people stick with most. Obviously, only what you continue to use will do you any good. A treadmill allows you to walk naturally at whatever pace you choose.

Caution: Be sure the speed can be set low enough for your comfortable starting pace. Also look for a model with good shock absorption, especially if you intend to jog. Start with *zero incline*—a slope can be hard on the back and neck. Some elderly people cannot get used to the "moving floor" and should consider a stationary bicycle.

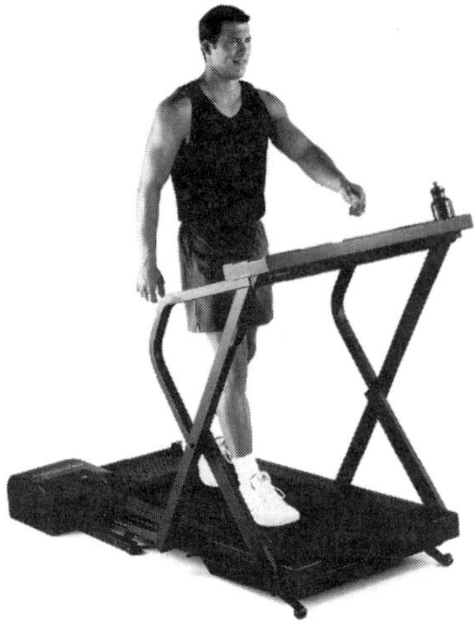

Photo of **ProForm** treadmill courtesy Icon Health & Fitness, Logan, Utah

Bicycling is best with minimum crouch (no swayed back) and legs nearly straight. A stationary exercise bicycle is convenient.

Jog with caution. Avoid hard impact. Use well-cushioned shoes and a running surface that gives. Look for imitation grass or other cushioning material. Jog with a tall posture and work up gradually.

Swimming. If your doctor approves, learn an endurance program and use it on a regular basis. Avoid the butterfly and breaststroke at least until you are pain free. The sidestroke is best for starting.

The Bottom Line

Neck pain almost always responds to the measures described in this booklet. Therefore, be hopeful. You must also be disciplined because there is no magic bullet. To become pain free and stay pain free, you may have to continue indefinitely with the program, watching your posture, doing stretching exercises, and following other recommendations. A modest price. A big reward.